Diabetic Guidebook

The Diabetics guide to delicious, healthy recipes and the most effective tips for combatting diabetes.

Table of Contents

Chapter 1 – Introduction

Diabetes no longer strikes terror into the hearts of the people who are plagued by it or by their loved ones because of the advanced scientific research and findings in the recent past. There are a number of ways in which this health condition can be dealt with but special emphasis is placed on the diet of the patient. For those of you who are unfamiliar with diabetes – it is a condition that causes insufficient production of insulin by the pancreas or when the body cells are not reacting well with the insulin produced. In many countries, this condition is also known as "having high blood sugar" or just "sugar". This is because when the insulin production and tolerance of the body is hampered, the level of glucose (commonly referred to as sugar) in the blood spikes or drops to irregular levels.

Although much advance has been made to deal with the worst aspects of this disease, there are still a number of precautions a person suffering from diabetes must take at all times to prevent or minimize diabetic attacks. Many patients lament at the stringent rules they have to follow about what they drink and eat. Food is one pleasure that man can savour at any time of the day in mind-boggling varieties. Any restrictions associated with food are usually severely detested because, admit it, we work really hard to earn our favourite meals and drinks. This book will primarily focus on what healthy and tasty options diabetic patients use to beat their hunger pangs without risking diabetic complications. The second part of the book will talk about the medical problems a diabetic would usually face because of unhealthy food practices so that you can avoid making these mistakes yourself.

Chapter 2 – Food for thoughts for diabetics!

A person suffering from diabetes or someone caring for a diabetic will freely admit that preparing a wholesome yet delicious meal under such circumstances is a real challenge. We know how difficult it may be for you to control natural urges and stop yourself from your favourite dishes because our doctor has deemed them unhealthy for you. Difficult as it may be, it is in your best interest to take heed to your doctor and steer clear of such dishes. What you could instead do is whip up one of the dishes in this book so that you can satisfy your hunger without taking any health risks at all!

Coming up next is a list of dishes and their recipes that we hope will make your fight against diabetes a little more nourished and tasty!

1. Tangy grilled chicken

Serves 4

Ingredients

- ¾ cup of lemon juice
- 4 chicken breasts cut in halves
- ¼ cup olive oil
- 1 tbsp thyme leaves
- 1 tsp salt
- Cooking spray

Method

In a Ziploc bag, mix well the chicken breasts, lemon juice, olive oil, thyme leaves and salt to marinate the chicken. Place the bag in fridge for an hour. You can keep turning the bag to evenly marinate the chicken pieces. Place the marinated chicken pieces on the grill rack, after you have removed the other items, and use the cooking spray on them. Grill each side on the chicken for at least 6 minutes, or until they are cooked, and then cut them slice them according to your choice.

To keep this dish interesting, what you can also do is prepare a salad that would go well with the chicken. Cooked peas, some bell pepper strips, a dash of cilantro, 1 tbsp. of olive oil, half cup of zucchini, 1 tsp. salt and a little bit of black pepper, all tossed together in a mixing bowl, sprinkled with the juice of 1-2 freshly squeezed lemons, will make a fabulous salad that will perfectly complement the grilled chicken.

2. Kebabs of vegetable and beefs served over rice

Serves 4

Ingredients

- 1 pound of boneless sirloin steak – wash well and preferably cut into cubes of 1" each.
- 8 mushrooms halved
- 1 large bell pepper cut into 1" pieces
- 2 green onions cut into 1" pieces – you should have about 8 such pieces
- 8 cherry or small tomatoes
- 1 tsp salt (kosher)
- ½ tsp of dried thyme
- 2 tsp of canola oil
- ¼ tsp of ground black pepper
- Cooking Spray

Method

The chopped and diced meat, mushrooms, bell pepper, green onions and tomatoes can be tossed together and then separated into 4 equal portions. Place each of these portions on a separate medium sized skewer (which is usually about 12" in width) and sprinkle over them the salt, thyme and black pepper. Place each of skewers one at a time on a broiling pan which has been pre-coated with cooking spray and sprinkle the kebabs with oil.

Broil the ingredients for about 10 minutes or until they have been cooked to your taste. Flip over the skewer once to allow all ingredients to be evenly cooked.

This preparation can be served with rice and is to be enjoyed hot, straight off the broiling pan.

3. A quiche of artichoke

Serves 6

Ingredients

- ¾ cup of reduced fat and sharp cheddar cheese that has been shredded and then separated
- 2 cups of cooked rice
- 1 tsp dried dillweed
- ¾ cup of egg substitute, also divided
- ½ tsp salt
- 1 tbsp of Dijon mustard
- ¼ tsp of freshly ground white pepper
- 1 garlic clove that has been crushed
- 1 can of artichoke hearts that have been quartered and then drained (1 can usually weighs about 14 ounce)
- ¼ cup of sliced green onions
- ¾ cup of fat-free milk
- Cooking spray

Strips of green onion can be used to be had with the dish but these are optional.

Method

This is best cooked in an oven. Pre-heat is to 350 degrees. While it is heating, put together the rice, ¼ cup of cheese, dillweed, salt, garlic and ¼ cup of the egg substitute. Take a pie-plate of about 9" and coat it with cooking spray. Press all these ingredients together in it. Place the tray in the oven and let the mixture cook for 5 minutes. This is part 1 of this dish and is for the preparation of the rice crust.

Take out the oven tray and place the quartered artichoke on a bottom of rice crust and sprinkle the rest of the cheese on it evenly. Mix the rest of the egg substitute, milk, Dijon mustard, sliced green onions and white pepper and pour the rest of the cheese on the mixture. Place this next in the even at the same temperature and let it cook for about 50 minutes. After that, remove the tray and let it cool for about 5 minutes. You can then cut the dish into wedges and have them with the green onion strips if you prefer to or enjoy them just like that. The rice crust makes this a very healthy option as compared to a pastry crust. The lack of excess sugar and meat makes this a very tasty and nutritious dish.

4. Balsamic fig sauce and chicken

Serves 4

Ingredients

- 4 boneless and skinless chicken breasts that have been halved
- ¾ cup of finely chopped onion
- ½ cup of fat free chicken broth which has less sodium content
- ¼ cup of balsamic vinegar
- 2 tsp of soy sauce, again with low sodium content
- ¼ cup of chopped dried figs
- 1.5 tbsp of fresh thyme leaves, separated
- 1 tbsp of olive oil
- 1 tbsp of butter
- ½ tsp of salt, divided

Method

Coat both sides of the chicken breasts with the thyme, salt and pepper. Make sure they are spread evenly. In a large non-stick skillet, heat the oil over medium-high heat and then add the coated chicken pieces. Cook each side for about 6 minutes or until they are done, flipping sides so both sides are evenly cooked. Remove the cooked chicken from the pan and keep it aside in a way it remains warm.

Reduce the heat now to medium and add butter to the pan. In it, add onion and sauté it for about 3 minutes. Add the rest of the ingredients – broth, vinegar, soy sauce and the chopped figs and let them cook well to make the sauce. Let this combination simmer so that the sauce can fit one cup which should take about 3-4 minutes. Add the thyme and salt to the sauce. This sauce can be had with the chicken breasts which have been halved or cut into slices. Pour the sauce on the cut chicken as they both taste well together.

5. Tuna steaks seared Mediterranean style

Serves 4

Ingredients

- 4 yellow fin tuna steaks each of about ¾" thickness
- 12 chopped and pitted kalamata olives
- 1 tbsp lemon juice
- 1 tbsp extra virgin olive oil
- 1.5 cups of chopped tomatoes
- ½ tsp of finely chopped garlic
- 1/8 tsp of ground coriander
- ½ tsp of salt
- ½ tsp of black pepper
- ¼ cup of green onions
- 1 tsp of drained capers
- 3 tbsp of parsley that has been chopped
- Cooking spray

Method

Take a large non-stick skillet and heat it on medium-heat flame. On the cut pieces of tuna, sprinkle salt, coriander and pepper evenly. The pan is to be coated with the cooking spray and in that place the coated fish. Cook each side of the fish for about 5 minutes or until it's been cooked to your taste preference.

In another pan, combine all the other ingredients you have, including the tomato, and create a fine paste; this should take about 4-5 minutes to be prepared in another small non-stick pan. When both dishes have been cooked, pour the tomato sauce over the seared fish and serve them hot.

6. Multigrain pulao

Serves 8

Ingredients

- ½ cup brown rice
- ½ cup uncooked barley (pearl)
- 2.5 cups of water
- 2 tsp Butter
- 1/3 cup of sunflower seed kernels
- 4 tsp of canola oil, divided
- ½ tsp salt, separated
- 1 cup of finely sliced leek (1 large leek should suffice for this)
- ½ cup of dried currants
- ¼ cup of uncooked bulgur
- ¼ cup of chopped parsley (fresh)
- ¼ tsp of fresh and ground pepper

Method

Medium-high heat a Dutch skillet. Add 2 tsps. Of oil, ¼ tsp. of salt and the sunflower seeds and sauté this mixture for about 2 minutes or until the seeds turn golden brown. Take the fried contents out and set it aside. Heat the same pan over medium heat and add the butter and the rest of the oil. While the oil and butter heat, add the chopped leek and cook it for about 4 minutes which should be sufficient enough to make it tender. Keep stirring the leek pieces else they will stick to the pan and get burnt. Once the leek is fried, add water and add the chicken broth, brown rice and pearl barley. Boil this entire mixture. When you see the contents in the pan bubbling, cover the pan, turn the gas flame to simmer and let them cook for the next 35 minutes. Thereafter, add the currants and bulgur and further simmer the contents for 10 minutes until all the items inside are tender. Take the pan off the stove, add the fried mixture that you had set aside and the rest of the salt and your dish is ready to be served, piping hot.

This is a wholesome and delicious dish that is also known as pilaf and pulav in certain parts of the world.

7. Walnuts and caramelized onions with green beans

Serves 5 (1 cup each)

Ingredients

- 1.5 pounds of trimmed green beans
- 1.2 cup of chopped walnuts
- 4 cups of onions that have been sliced thin and vertically
- 2 tbsp of extra virgin olive oil, divided
- 1 tsp of fresh thyme, chopped
- 2 tsp of balsamic vinegar
- ¼ tsp of freshly ground black pepper
- ½ tsp of kosher salt

Method

Place the chopped beans in a pan and pour sufficient water to let them all boil fully. This should take about 2-3 minutes. Once boiled, drain the hot water, rinse the beans with cold water and then drain that water too. Place the boiled beans aside. Next, take a large non-stick skillet and set it over medium heat. Pour the chopped walnuts in the pan and heat them until they turn light brown. Keep shaking the pan so that the walnuts don't group together and get burnt and to ensure they are all browned equally. Once the walnuts are lightly fried, remove them from the pan and keep them aside. In the same pan, add 4 tsps. Of oil and swirl it so that it covers the complete diameter of the pan base. Add the chopped onions and thyme to the heating oil and cook for about 17 minutes so that the onion strips are very tender and get a golden brown hue. Keep stirring the pan as you did for the walnuts. Take out the caramelized onions and keep them aside too.

Place the same pan again on medium-high heat and add the remaining olive oil in the pan. Swirl the pan again to ensure the oil is evenly spread. Now, add the green beans and cook until they are completely heated which should be done in about 2 minutes. Add the onion strips and vinegar to the pan and cook for another 2 minutes. While they are getting cooked, keep tossing the ingredients so they all get cooked well and the onions remain crispy but not burnt. Take the pan off the heat, add the fried walnuts and our delicious dish is ready to be served.

8. Black Beans and Quinoa

Serves 2

Ingredients

- 3 tbsp of quinoa, separated
- ¼ cup and 2 tsps of vegetable broth
- ¼ onion, minced well
- ¼ tsp of vegetable oil
- ¼ tsp of ground cumin
- 1/8 tsp of cayenne pepper
- 15 ounces of black beans (which is about 3/8 of a can), rinsed and drained
- 5/8 cloves of garlic, finely chopped
- 3.5 tbsp of frozen corn kernels, separated
- 3 tsp of fresh cilantro, finely chopped
- Salt and ground black pepper as per taste

Method

Take a medium sized saucepan and heat the oil in it over medium heat. Add garlic and onion and cook them until they turn light brown. This should take about 10 minutes. Add quinoa to the pan and then add the vegetable broth. To this bubbling mixture, add the seasonings of cumin, salt, pepper and cayenne pepper. Cook until the mixture starts boiling. Once it starts boiling, turn down the flame to low-medium and cover to let the mixture simmer. Let it simmer until the quinoa becomes soft and the broth is absorbed completely; this should be done in about 20 minutes. Take the cover off and add the corn to the pan, continue to let the mixture simmer on the same heat for about 5 minutes. In the end, add the cilantro and black beans. Take it off the stove and serve hot.

9. Tomato, peas and chicken

Serves 5

Ingredients

- 5 boneless and skinless chicken breasts, halved (6 ounces)
- 1 can of chopped tomatoes (16 ounces)
- 1 tsp basil
- 2 tbsp of diced garlic
- 2 tbsp of soy sauce
- 1 tbsp dry mustard
- ½ packet of frozen peas (10 ounces)

Method

This dish requires a slow cooker to thoroughly cook the chicken breasts and frozen peas. So in a slow cooker, add the chicken breasts and let it cook slowly. At the same time, take a pan and add tomatoes, basil, dry mustard, garlic and to sauce to make a paste. Pour the paste on the chicken in the slow cooker and let them cook together. This mixture will have to be kept in the cooker for 7 hours to allow it to cook fully. After 7 hours, add the frozen peas and let it all cook for another hour. At the end of the 8th hour, when the chicken and peas are tender (fully cooked), take the cooker off the stove and serve the dish hot.

10.   Rice with black beans

Serves 10

Ingredients

- 3.5 cups of black beans, drained
- 1.5 cups of low sodium and low fat vegetable broth
- ¾ cup of white rice, uncooked
- 1 tsp olive oil
- 1 large onion, chopped finely
- 2 garlic cloves, finely chopped

- 1 tsp cumin powder
- ¼ tsp cayenne pepper

Method

Place a deep pot over medium-high flame and pour the oil. After the oil has heated, add the chopped onion and garlic cloves and sauté for about 4 minutes. Next, add the uncooked rice and sauté for another 2 minutes. To this mixture, add the vegetable broth and bring them all to boil. When the mixture starts bubbling, cover it and bring the heat down to low. Let the mixture simmer for about 20 minutes. Add all the spices and black beans and then serve the dish hot.

11.   Curry of red lentil

Serves 8

Ingredients

- 2 cups of red lentil
- 1 large onion, chopped fine
- 1 tbsp vegetable oil
- 2 tbsp Curry paste
- 1 tbsp curry powder
- 1 tsp salt
- 1 tsp sugar (white)
- 1 tsp fresh ginger (minced)
- 1 tsp chilli powder
- 1 tsp finely minced garlic
- 1 tsp cumin
- 1 tsp turmeric powder
- 1 can of tomato puree (about 14 ounce)

Method

The lentils must be washed in cold water until the water poured out becomes clear. Place the thoroughly washed and drained lentils in a pot which should be sufficient to also hold enough water for cooking. Bring the water and lentils mixture to boil and then place a cover over it. Turn down the flame from high to medium-low and let the mixture simmer. Keep adding water in between to let the lentils become soft. This should take about 15-20 minutes. Drain this mixture. Next, place a skillet on medium heat and pour the vegetable oil in it. Add the chopped onions and cook until they caramelize. This should take about 20 minutes. In a separate bowl, mix the curry powder, curry paste, cumin, chilli powder, turmeric, sugar, salt, garlic and ginger and add this mixture to the caramelized onions. Turn the heat to high and cook this mixture for 1-2 minutes until it starts giving out a fragrance. To this, add the tomato puree and remove it after 1-2 minutes. Pour this over the lentils and serve the dish hot. This is best consumed with flattened bread (rotis) or rice which should also be hot.

12.   Meatloaf of vegetables

Serves 8

Ingredients

- 1 bottle of barbeque sauce (12 ounce)
- 1 packet of vegetarian burger crumbles (12 ounce)
- 1 green bell pepper, diced
- 1/3 cup of finely chopped onion
- 1 garlic clove, minced
- ½ cup of softened bread crumbs
- 1 beaten egg
- 2 tbsp of Parmesan cheese
- ¼ tsp dried thyme
- ¼ tsp dried basil
- Salt and pepper according to taste
- ¼ tsp of parsley flakes

Method

Preheat the oven to 165 degrees C (325 degrees F). In this, place a lightly greased loaf pan measuring 5x9. Take a bowl and mix half the barbeque sauce, vegetarian burger crumbles, onion, garlic, green bell pepper, parmesan cheese, egg and the softened bread crumbs. Add the seasonings of basil, thyme, pepper, salt and parsley. Let this mixture cook for about 5 minutes and then transfer it to the oven loaf pan. Leave it in the oven for 40 minutes. After that, add the rest of the barbeque sauce on the loaf and let it cook for another 15 minutes or until the loaf sets. Take out from oven and serve hot.

Chapter 3 –Health care for diabetics

People who have diabetes should be extra cautious about their daily habits to prevent diabetic complications. As this is one of those diseases that tend to develop in people after they have hit a certain age, they are likely to be accompanied by other problems such as cardiac issues and blood pressure irregularities. If one of these problems becomes more serious, the other health conditions also worsen at the same time.

It has also been noted that people cannot be treated for disease as well as they could have been because another health complication prevents doctors from doing so. For example, if a person suffers a cardiac arrest, doctors may want to do a particular kind of heart surgery which will yield the best results. But because the patient has a history of diabetes and may not be able to recover from the surgery completely, the doctors may opt against that procedure and instead choose another one which may be enough to just keep the patient alive but the problem doesn't get solved completely.

Diabetics are also known to be poor healers. They take longer to recover from surgeries; their wounds take a long time to heal. Even small cuts remain raw and painful for a longer time in such people. Many people have such severe diabetes they have to treat themselves with insulin shots! So rather than facing all these complications, there are a few changes to your lifestyle that you can make and easily keep diabetes under control. Here are a few of them.

1. **Make up your mind** – Managing diabetes requires a lot of self-control. You must remember that there are certain activities you cannot do and more importantly, there are foods and drinks that you cannot consume. You may want to indulge in them occasionally but you should avoid them at all costs because they will certainly cause your blood sugar levels to rise to dangerous and sometimes fatal levels. It is important that you consult your doctor and fitness experts from time to time to know what are the best medicines, precautionary measures and low-key exercises that you can do to manage diabetes. When you get a level of self-control, share your problems with health professionals and get adequate

informative support, your mind can easily overcome temptations and will be fully aware of all the problems that you may face. When your mind is set, you can easily follow all the remaining steps.

2. **Quit smoking** – After food and drinking, smoking is perhaps one habit that is extremely common and is very, very hard to give up. There is dark joke about smoking that you may have heard – I think of quitting smoking but in order to think, I light another cigarette. Cigarette and any other form of smoking is unhealthy for everyone, it has zero health benefits. But for a diabetic, they are especially harmful and must be avoided at all costs. Here are just some of the ways in which smoking affects a person:

   a. It reduces the healthy supply of blood to all parts of the body which causes health complications like ulcers, gangrene and infections which do not heal due to diabetes. Since those body parts cannot be healed, those parts are often removed (amputated) from the body. So smoking can cost you one or more limbs in the long run.
   b. They increase heart diseases.
   c. You have higher chances of suffering from a stroke.
   d. They cause nerve damages.
   e. They could lead to eye diseases which could lead to blindness
   f. They can cause kidney related diseases' complication.

3. **Regulate your blood pressure and cholesterol levels** – As mentioned earlier, these additional diseases become more complicated due to diabetes and cannot be treated as easily. They damage several organs (at the cells and tissue levels) and thus become very hard to detect initially and be treated early on. Even blood vessels can be damaged due to high blood pressure. If you maintain a healthy, low fat and low sodium diet and if you exercise regularly, you can keep all these conditions under control.

4. **Be vaccinated and hygienic** – One of the side-effects of being diabetic is that your immune system doesn't work optimally, thus making it susceptible to many kinds of diseases. You may be one of those who are always plagued by flu, aches and allergies if you

don't take adequate precautions against their stimulants. One way to do so is be extremely hygienic and keep your environment clean. Another way of warding off diseases is by using only your cleaning paraphernalia (such as wet wipes, kerchiefs, combs and towels) when you want to clean yourself up; avoid using personal articles of other people. The third preventive measure you can use is to always keep a hand sanitizer with you. Use it frequently so that your hands remain germ-free.

Get appropriate vaccinations. Diabetics should especially be aware of the vaccines they must take and how often they should get vaccinations. Some of the vaccines that prove useful are those for flu, pneumonia, Hepatitis B and tetanus shots.

5. **Dental care** – We are all aware that the teeth and gums are storehouses of many bacteria if they are not brushed properly and regularly. These cause many problems such as malodour and teeth pain. But for diabetics, treating them becomes very problematic. These are issues that happen in a closed part of the body which in itself delays the healing process. Add diabetes to the combination and you will see that they take an even longer and painful time to heal. So maintain good dental hygiene by including mouthwash rinsing and flossing in your regular routine. Pay attention to the colour of your teeth and the health of your gums. And most importantly, visit your dentist for a check-up at least twice a year so that they can spot any dental problems.

6. **Feet hygiene** –Just like your teeth, even the webs of your feet and toe nails have several micro-organisms hidden in them because these are parts of the body that we don't take adequate care of. If you have diabetes and suffer wounds, lesions or even minor scratches, do not take them lightly and leave them unattended. As mentioned earlier, these take a very long amount of time to heal which encourages further attacks from bacteria and virus to the affected portions thus leading to the rotting of those parts. If these parts cannot be healed, they will have to be cut off or those parts will have to be treated with such high-strength medicines that you lose all feelings in those parts. In order to keep your feet hassle-free, here are some tips for you:

a. Instead of washing your feet with cold water or soaking them for long periods of time in hot water, use lukewarm water to wash all parts of your feet. Using very hot water may lead to excessively dry feet.

b. After you wash your feet, dry them gently with a soft and clean towel or with medically treated wet wipes.

c. Keep your feet supple by using moisturisers, petroleum jelly or lotions. Dry feet get bruised and cut easier than moisturised feet. But be careful to not over-use these products and avoid using them in the feet webs as they may lead to growth of bacteria.

d. Be sure to check your feet every day for any fresh cuts or bruises so you can treat them immediately. Blisters, sores, swelling and redness too should be treated carefully.

7. **Control your drinking habits** – It would be helpful if you avoid drinking altogether but if you cannot do so, then you should make sure you drink in a responsible manner. Avoid drinks with high alcoholic percentages and opt for the milder drinks. Alcoholic drinks too have calories, do remember they too add to your daily calories count and have an impact on your heart and blood pressure. Do not drink on an empty stomach but have a drink after you have had your meal.

8. **Avoid stress** – Stress is another factor that triggers diabetic attacks. Stress leads to improper functioning of our body glands and organs. As insulin is also produced by an organ, stress leads to irregular supple of insulin thus acting as a direct diabetic factor. Learn to avoid problematic situations, stress controlling techniques such as breathing exercises, meditation and yoga, sleep for an adequate number of hours every day and set limits on how much you let a person or incident impact you.

Conclusion

Out of all the tactics you use to maintain diabetes, maintaining your diet is the most important one because your food habits directly impact your cholesterol and blood pressure levels, impact stress handling capacity, ensure the supply of blood is adequate and even, prevents obesity and keeps all internal organs working smoothly. Most of the recipes mentioned in this book are high on protein content and exclude fat completely.

You would have also noticed the inclusion of plenty of herbs and spices that we generally don't include in our daily dishes. Non-starchy and green vegetables should take up the lion's share of your dinner plate, followed by a small portion of grains and starchy foods such as rice, pasta and oatmeal. Next, include proteins in your diet by adding a portion of meat which has been completely de-skinned. Also include fish as an alternative to meat at least twice a week. Next, add a portion of fruits and milk products (the latter only if you don't have any milk-related allergies) in your diet in the form of desserts. Try and have whole fruits as much as possible instead of relying on their juices or squashes. Finally, pay attention to the oil that you use to cook. Try avoiding fatty oils and instead opt for olive oil as much as possible. Also include as much seeds and nuts in your diet (again keeping in mind any allergies you may have towards them) and you've got yourself a balanced meal plan that will help you not only with diabetes but with all other health-related problems.

When you maintain a balanced diet and have an active life, diabetes takes a backseat and you can enjoy life to its fullest. So try some of the recipes listed here or look for similar ones and get started with beating diabetes today.

www.ingramcontent.com/pod-product-compliance
Lightning Source LLC
Chambersburg PA
CBHW081145280526
45787CB00007B/3229